The SCENT of ANGELS

Front Lines of Barbed Wire

This book was written 5 years Before
WAR HORSE iN Book & Film lied the Media
This is a true event of war Horses page 51
lived & died.

Best wishes

Margaret Le Grange

The SCENT of ANGELS

Front Lines of Barbed Wire

Margaret Le Grange

First published 2016

A CIP catalogue record for this book is available
from the British Library

ISBN 978 0 9932988 3 7

Contact Margaret by writing to:

Margaret Le Grange
Guide Light Cottage
38 Boscaswell Village
Pendeen, Penzance
Cornwall TR19 7EP

Cover illustration by the Author

Printed in Great Britain by Booksprint

Preface

These are short biographies as given to me over a period of five years. They are recorded in long hand, through clairvoyance and speed writing.

As with **Battlefield Memories** and **Lest We Forget** I see the world of events through their eyes – life in the trenches; when the bullets hit; being blown into bits in an aeroplane, or drowning in the sea, all in the blink of an eye. Taste, smell, noise – I hear them all but I can release myself from it all.

The stories are taken down word for word, nothing is changed: only the grammar and spelling is corrected so it is easier to read.

Contents

		Foreword	9
		Preface – Lest We Forget	11
1.	1914	Foot Soldier	13
2.	1914	Shot at Dawn	17
3.	1914	German Medical Corporal	19
4.	1915	Tobias	21
5.	1915	Gassed	23
6.	1916	I foresaw my Death	27
7.	1916	Belgium School Master	29
8.	1916	First Battalion of Lancers	31
9.	1916	Canadian Soldier	33
10.	1917	Cuthbert's Story	37
11.	1917	The Shepherd (1 and 2)	39
12.	1917	Harry…War Animals	42
13.	1917	Coal Miner	44
14.	1917	Spotter Plane	46
15.	1906-1922	H.M.S.Dreadnought	48
16.	1940	Henry	51
17.	1940	Dog Fight for Britain	52
18.	1940	Hurricane	54
19.	1941	H.M.S. Hood	56
20.	1941	Bismark	58
21.	1943	Hell Fire Pass	62
22.	1943	Gurkha Soldier	66
23.	1944	Regrets	69
24.	1944	Hospital Ship	73

As given to Margaret Le Grange, Psychic Biographer

Foreword

Finally, in our 21st century, the paranormal becomes acceptable and mainstream. Margaret Le Grange has the privilege of hearing messages from Beyond, and she transmits them to us in a style that flows and sparkles like a Dartmoor stream.

This collection contains many accounts from the two major world wars in the last century, stretching from Ceylon to Canada.

Fundamentally, these stories can be read at three levels – the historic, the personal, and the supernatural.

Details of the wars and major events are narrated here. Souls present poignant accounts of their background, their reasons for going to war, their emotions, the nitty-gritty of the trenches (WW1), the courage they employed in those aeroplanes, sinking ships (WW2) and much more.

The full gamut of human experience lies within these pages, from youthful enthusiasm and valour, right through the pain, the fear, the torment, the heroic feats, the the moment of Death and beyond. Yet, these men and women, now long departed from this world, still possess refreshing memories of home life, loving families, their homeland. There are passages of breath-taking beauty as well as moments of sheer horror. Not even the horses are spared, sharing the mud and the squalor of the trenches with the humans.

The supernatural – the passage of one state of being to another is depicetd in various ways by different souls, affording us an insight into that world of mystery and awe, Death and glimpses of the Afterlife.

I have nothing but praise and admiration for Margaret Le Grange – she writes it all down effortlessly, with grace and poignancy. The end result is a most readable and enlightening book.

Dulce Pombeiro
Lecturer and Translator
July 2009

Lest We Forget 1914-2009

Let us cast our minds back to the 1914-1918 War.

Recently the last Tommy, Harry Patch, passed away aged 111 years old. Bless his soul. There was no media television or radio coverage on that bloody slaughter of our young men taken in the prime of life, some barely twenty years of age. Most were forced to join up but some went willingly, taking the King's Shilling which was the most money some would ever see in their lives.

No day to day images were shown of soldiers marching or lying dead in mud-filled trenches, or animals, horses, dogs and pigeons – pets sent by their owners. A racehorse beautifully cared for, children's beloved ponies, sent with the promise they would be returned when the war ended.

Did they return? No. Those who did survive suffered so badly from their wounds and shell shock that the MOD sold them cheaply to Egypt as working beasts to carry unbearably heavy loads and some animals were eaten. Not one horse came back to England: did you know this? The rare letter stating that "Your son, brother, husband is missing, presumed dead" was all that the generation got. The dead were never sent home to be buried in England's soil. What horrors and torment they must have suffered!

One news reporter recently said, after Harry Patch had died: "Well, that's the end of World War I. No more first hand knowledge will ever be known" as if to say that that chapter is closed.

If that generation had news like relatives have today, do you think that Britain would have gone into World War II? Of course not. Although in WWII information was more readily available about the war which was spread over Europe and the Far East, still no one got their loved ones back to bury and to mourn.

Now, I think, there is much too much media coverage of the personal side of wars today with pictures of sons, brothers, fathers appearing on most news reports. My heart goes out to the families of each young man but I believe grief is private. Most people must appreciate that war of any kind causes devastation on all sides.

Let us remember all those still missing from 1914-1918 – 100,000 unaccounted for young men, and the families who, perhaps, still hope for news.

At the going down of the sun and in the morning, we shall remember them.

Margaret Le Grange

Foot Soldier

"I'm over here. I'm a corporal and a foot soldier, serving with the Devon and Somerset Regiment.

We came over in August 1914 when the war was just starting. I was 24 years old and my name is Wilfred. I lived in Exeter and was one of the first men to join at the beginning of the war.

I was married and left behind a lovely wife, Nancy, and three children: my eldest, a girl named Lucy, a boy, Edward, and a baby but a few weeks old, not yet named.

I was tall, of slender build, fair-haired with brown eyes. I wore no badge of rank, just the name of my regiment. Just one of hundreds of foot soldiers who did all the fighting. My uniform was khaki trousers, tucked into spats and boots, carrying my kit bag and my new rifle. Sometimes we wore coarse netting stretched over our metal helmets to give us camouflage when in the trenches…

We had faced some terrible front line fighting and time was running out for our regiment while waiting for reinforcements to come up the line.

Our wireless operator kept sending messages calling for SOS, requesting back-up from the Royal Scottish Sutherland Highlanders, under the command of General McAllister. They were bogged down in Flanders mud: the horses could not pull the gun carriages and the men had to pull and push them. Hence the critical delay and they didn't get to us in time for the big push forward to make a joint advancement as planned over the barbed wire front lines. If we had had their support, we would not have suffered such a great loss.

The Highlanders' motto was *No Prisoners.* They were magnificent fighters dressed in their national uniform, white spats and swishing kilts, played into battle by their pipe major on the bagpipes. You could hear them coming but this day there was no sound of bagpipes: we were straining our ears to hear.

What a bloody slaughter it was. We were virtually wiped out. I never saw another sun set or another dawn. I had a clean kill straight through my heart. One moment I was running, head down, bayonet fixed. I had done this a couple of times before and returned safely, now I would never see my comrades again, or so I thought. The world stood still: it was silent and as I fell in slow motion and buried my face in the mud in No Man's Land, I had the sensation of hands lifting me up. At that moment I did not know that I was dead. How could I, as I had never had an experience like this before.

No more pain, no mud or stench of the dead, just a host of light beings, not angels, as they had no wings, which I would have recognised from the bedtime stories told to me as a child of a very strict Roman Catholic family. My father was an objector and would not fight. His very last words to me were: *Son, if you kill anyone, you will live in Hell for Eternity.* He was wrong: this was not Hell, it was beautiful. Hell was on Earth in the trenches, but he would not have known this.

God bless you, my friend, for sharing a moment of your time with me. I died on The Somme on an August day, a few days after I went into battle in 1914.

If the artillery reinforcements had come in time perhaps I might have lived longer. But time was of the essence and the generals did not take into account the mud or how important our lives were to all of us. It was not my war but that of the officers. They gave us the orders but did not follow us over the top."

Received: August 2006

I went to see the soldiers

I went to see the soldiers, row on row on row,
And wondered about each so still, their badges all on show.
What brought them here, what life before
Was like for each of them?

These soldiers, boys and men.
Some so young, some older still, a bond more close than brothers
These men have earned and shared a love, that's not like any others
They trained as one, they fought as one
They shared their last together
That bond endures, that love is true
And will be now and ever.

I could not know, how could I guess, what choices each had made,
Of how they came to soldiering, what part each one had played?
But here they are and here they'll stay,
Each one silent and in place,
Their headstones line up row on row
They guard this hallowed place.

Kenny Martin

The Paper Dove

Its soft white feathers flutter in the wind,
Gliding gently over fields
And countries torn by war,
It has no idea of the fighting below,

Its soft white feathers flutter in the wind,
Its eyes are heavy,
Visions lie heavy in its mind,
The poppy fields glide past,

Its soft white feathers flutter in the wind,
They feel the blasts,
The pain,
The black mass that engulfs the men,

Its soft white feathers flutter in the wind,
Children crying for their fathers,
After reading letters of loss,
The endless sombre parades,

Its soft white feathers flutter in the wind,
Love lies underneath,
Blood red poppies scattered below,
The folded feathers float onto the poppy fields.

Its soft white feathers flutter in the wind,
Launched by a child, off mountains high,
Watched by millions,
A peace spreader,
A hope bringer,
Only soft white paper feathers fall in the wind,
From The Paper Dove.

Mark aged 14

Shot at Dawn, at the Somme, 1914

"Hallo, my friend: I've come today to tell you of my brief moment on this earth.

My name is Howard and I'm just 17 and a half years old. I looked older than I really was… I joined up with my buddy, Thomas, who was a few months older than me. We were told that a war was coming and being young with no fear we thought, *shall we go and have an adventure?* Never for one moment thinking of the dangers we were going to face. Thousands of young boys and men joined up a few weeks after the beginning of the war.

It was September 1914 when a dream turned into a nightmare...

We were rushed through the fundamental rules of war, how to shoot your rifle and hit the target you were aiming for, and, most of all, the vital importance of keeping your rifle clean as your life might depend on it.

Then we were on a ship, crossing the Channel to Normandy, the days of marching, carrying your heavy kit bag which got heavier with each mile we marched. At first the roads were very much like England's with flowers along the hedgerows, but as we moved further inland and came across where the fighting had taken place, the pretty countryside became sinister, and sad.

This is when Thomas and I thought, *O God, what have we done?* But there was no going back, war signs were all around us. On the third day we came across what looked like enormous earthworks known as trenches. They did not run in straight lines, but everywhere. This was going to be our home for the rest of our lives. No one knew how long it would be in this rat-ridden hole in the ground. It was the first time I had ever seen anyone dead, but it would not be the last.

I come from Ross on Wye in Herefordshire. I never got further than the end of our road, not even to the next village. Now we were looking on a vast sea of mud, the bloated bodies of horses and men, flies and the stench of death which made me gag and be sick. It was utterly appalling: why had someone not buried them? It was so cold. I think the coldness was the fear we felt. Mam would be horrified if she knew where her little son was… A flash of childhood days: pranks; scrumping Mr. Jones's apples; climbing walls, and shinning up trees. That was fun: this was not fun anymore…

Thomas said: *We might as well put a brave face on it. There's no turning back now. We might be lucky.* But we had no idea what lay ahead of us.

My first night I was on duty as watchman, a sentry. I stared unblinking into the dark night, heard some faint song being sung, smelt food being cooked. After marching all day, I fought to keep my eyes open as sleep swept over me. But I knew that I could not go to sleep. I kept shaking my head and biting my bottom lip to keep awake but sleep finally overtook me and I closed my eyes just for a second.

A sharp crack in my ribs, swearing enough to waken the dead: no excuses allowed. I was arrested and marched off. It was the end of the war for me. I was tied to a post by my arms and a tie put around my knees, blind folded.

I heard Thomas's voice and he laid down his rifle and refused to shoot and kill his buddy. A lot of shouting took place. I could not see what was going on but he was court martialled, tied to a post beside me and we were both shot at 4.30am. My crime was for being asleep on duty and Tom's for disobeying an order.

In hindsight they could not really afford to kill their own men as there were too few already. But discipline was a prime ruling.

So ended our short lives, side by side, on a misty September morning, the 29th, 1914. Neither of us had fired a shot, murdered by our own men, felled by friendly fire. It was not friendly, neither of us had a grave but were rolled into a shallow hollow in the field where we were shot, never to be found to this day...

Rules were made up on the field: it must be shown that we were cowards and must be shown as a warning to the rest of the men.

Mother received a letter (she could not read) stating that her son was shot as a coward. Thomas's mam killed herself with the shame of it. I was not a coward. I closed my eyes for a second, but was not asleep.

Thank you for listening to me and writing down my story. I was the eldest of four children. I should have stayed at home to look after the family but the thought of adventure was too exciting."

Howard was a small lad with brown hair and grey eyes set into a thin, narrow face. His teeth were uneven. He tells me his nickname was Howie. Thomas was a little taller with black hair and grey-green eyes. He had a large gap between his front teeth.

Received: 05/01/2007

18

German Medical Corporal

My name is Wolfgang. I am 17 years old, serving with the German Light Infantry.

I work as a medical assistant but also I have to bring in our wounded soldiers. There are four of us. The ones under me are orderlies of no special rank. Usually the walking injured are used for this task. The injured are brought to me: if I can feel a pulse, I admit them. No pulse, we put them to one side for burial at the end of the day...

Our field hospital is mostly a large tent or sometimes we commandeer a house or barn behind our front lines out of reach of the Tommies' guns.

Firstly, the stretchers are laid out in rows out of the ever increasing rain which does not stop. I say to myself, *God is weeping* for this war, brother against brother, that's why it rains so much.

When a canvas cot is available, the wounded are brought in, usually the worst first. Our surgeon is good with the saw. There are many legs and so much blood on the floor... It is quicker to cut off the leg than to mend it.

On one trip, a young British boy was brought in, mistaken for one of ours. I felt his pulse, he opened his eyes and called for his mutter (mother). I did not have the heart to turn him away so put him in a spare cot. At that moment the officer came in. He spotted the lad and took out his pistol to kill him. He said *No prisoners* and put his pistol to his head. There was so much blood on this young face. I stepped forward to shield his body and I put my hand on the pistol saying, *Is not his blood the same colour as yours? Has he not got the same chance as our boys?* He clicked his heels together, scowled at me and said, *You will be reported for this.*

I called after him, saying, *Do you not think the British would not treat one of ours if the situation was the same?*

I held his hand and wiped his small face clean of blood. He asked many times for his mother. He was so much like my little brother back home. He said that his name was Michael and he was 17 years old.

I, as a Christian, said a prayer for him as he died on the first day of September 1914.

I was killed, also shot in the head, a few days later on the third, but I had no one to hold my hand or say a prayer over me.

My home was in Freiburg in the Black Forest. We are glad of kind people like you to help heal the wounds of war.

Tobias

Hello, I am Tobias, called Toby by my friends.

Firstly, let me tell you about my name. It's not a typical English name as I am of mixed blood, but of course it does not matter up here but in England it was looked on as Trouble and despised by all the Whites even as far back as the 1900s. My grandmother was born in Trinidad while under British rule. She was married to a white man and from that time everyone was white but I inherited the Trinidad black, curly hair.

Now that I have that said, I will continue with my life as it was up to the time of my death in 1915.

During my youth I ran wild, too many in the family to really care about one little boy. I stole everything and sold it on, giving myself a reputation which followed me into the army in 1914.

I moved away from London. Work was easy to find if you were able to work and did not mind the work. Of course, stealing and not being caught was better. At first I supported my family but soon tired of that, finally ending up in Nottingham when the war broke out. At 17, circumstances forced me to join up, to avoid the law.

So, along with hundreds of others, I took the King's Shilling and went to war. I joined the Light Infantry of the Sherwood Foresters, landing on Dutch soil in late September 1915. I was just 17.

What a rude awakening it was. It was a bloody war and the first day casualties were the heaviest of the war for one single day. It devastated the morale of the British back home. So many foot soldiers and officers and horses died that first day. The British Army was not really ready in any way to cope with what the Germans threw at them. We were badly equipped: our weapons were poor and there were many faults. The uniforms were inadequate and the boots were dreadful. We had not got the fire power, mortars and machine guns, like the Germans had. It was bloody slaughter. I found all this out after my death.

Most generals went to war riding on horses as if they were going out for a weekend of pheasant shooting.

The countryside was not damaged: wild flowers grew in hedgerows and trenches were still being dug in rock-hard clay. The rains had not yet come. The countryside was not ravaged by war. But when it started to rain, the trenches filled up with water as the heavy clay would not let it drain away.

As I said, I was able to get anything, so I stole a chicken here and there, and apples from the now standing deserted orchards, and soon I was called upon to get other things. The word got around: *Ask Toby: he will get it.*

Our front lines were made of barbed wire which we had to make our way through on every attack we made. We were all terrified of going over the top but we had no choice. To refuse to go would mean you were a coward and you would be shot by our own men. None of us knew which bullet had our name on it. I never felt my bullet: it happened so fast.

When the mortars were whizzing over, you could not hear the birds but now, all of a sudden, I was in a different world. It was so quiet and bright and I could hear the birds singing. I seemed to be all on my own at first: there were no trenches of mud, no smell of gun fire, but quiet, bright, and it seemed to me I could actually hear the grass growing. I was not frightened but more amazed, then more of my comrades joined me. I felt like singing; I could not take it all in. I did not know that I was dead then.

Then I heard my name being called but all I could see was hundreds of children, all colours and ages. What were they doing on a battlefield? They came and took us by the hand, running, pulling us along to follow them.

I am glad I made contact with you today: it explains it all so clearly now, thank you. I first appeared to you just as you were coming out of sleep. Spirit tells me that this is the best way to contact you, it's easier this way, when all your senses are relaxed.

Tobias…Toby   30th September 1915

Received March 2009

Gassed 1915

Hallo, my name is Dick. I was serving with the Lancashire Regiment. Mam died at my birth along with my little sister aged two years old. Papa died tragically a month after I was born, run down by a horse and cart. I don't know any more than this, and all too soon, memories like this are blotted out in my young memory.

My grandparents brought me up and they had a nickname for me as Barley Boy as it was the colour of my hair. Grandpa said the colour of my hair was like the ripening of barley so that name stuck with me the whole of my life. I had a happy life with them. When grandma talked about me, she would say: *He is my Barley Boy! So much like his father at this age.* It was a very loving home and I loved them dearly, as the only parents I knew. They retired a few years after I joined their family, both of them in their sixties but I did not lack for anything.

Grandpa had owned and run a grocery store, and they had a lovely old house set off the lane by large trees. Grandma had brought up six boys and two girls. Now she had a baby in the house again. Like a mother hen, she fussed around me. I remember the garden as I grew up: trees to climb and well-kept lawns and flowers of every colour, and an old bee hive always busy with bees. I was woken every morning by the blackbird singing.

Now I was in a different world. I had joined up for an adventure like all my school pals in 1915. I left school at 13 and became a delivery boy. So at the age of 17, I was ready to spread my wings: the Lancashire Regiment gave me that chance. Grandma did not want me to go but they did nothing to stop me. I wish I had heeded them now but it was too late.

I thought I knew it all and was head strong. This war was not going to last long. I would soon be home again.

I was excited, carried along on the wave of gossip. It was not until we walked off the boat onto the Dutch coast that we all realised what we had done. No going back now. Fear hung around me like a wet blanket, chilling me to the bone and to my utter soul.

We marched through small villages torn apart by war. Derelict houses broken and smashed by canon fire. Timid folk standing, waving us by, with the hope that the Tommies had come to save them. How flat this land was: no trees, but strange buildings with arms. I was told that they were windmills. A lot of deep ditches, of water between the fields, all so unlike England. It was, indeed, a very strange land. It seemed to rain a lot.

It was autumn now. My homeland would be a blaze of burning colours, but here, not a sign of colour: it all looked dreary and tired. We were exhausted when we billeted in a barn to sleep the night. Rations were issued in our metal dishes and hot, sweet tea was very welcome. The night was damp as we lay cheek by jowl in any space we could find, leaving our boots on for fear rats. This would be the last dry night most of us would know.

We were a replacement regiment as the first wave of British soldiers had taken a great loss of manpower in the first months of the war. Conditions were appalling, much worse than we had been prepared for. The officers never told us the truth, or what lay ahead. Our equipment was sparse: rifle and bayonet kit bag and a trench coat. It was made of a heavy material which we were grateful for as it kept out the rain and kept us warm. We had a bed roll which was little use, we later found out.

Fear broke out among the ranks as the young ones faced the reality of how appalling the actual situation was. The trenches were full of stinking water, the dead and huge rats. We could not understand why the dead just lay there where they fell and were not taken away and buried. I learnt that after the fighting the men were too tired to do anything but sit and sleep, those that came back alive.

We were told that the Germans had started to use gas which would float across the front lines in clouds. Unfortunately the British were not prepared for the gas: in fact, they had no protection for us. The only hope we had was to urinate on a piece of cloth and tie it over our mouths and nose but it gave no protection to our eyes. In 1915 the British Tommies died like flies without adequate protection from gas attacks.

This is where I got it, in a gas attack. It was impossible to urinate when everyone was panicking when clouds of sulphur-yellow gas came drifting into our trenches. A warning was meant to be given but often it would come too late. It was by a shout, GAS! But if were not within earshot you would not know to urinate on your rag which the army issued us with.

Soon after we arrived there was a lull in the fighting and we were able to catch up with news from the Front. I later found a small place to sit, awaiting the arrival of the evening meal. As I sat quietly, my thoughts were on home: would I ever see it again? It was then that I heard the small voice of my sister call my name: she always came to me during my childhood to warn me of a danger. Now she said: *Dick: hear me. Your time out here is going to be short but I will always be at your side. You are not alone. I will take you home.* The presence that I felt was gone. I never told anyone at home about Mary as it was my secret and I was always so happy that she had found me here in this awful place.

I had no idea how short that the time was going to be. It was about three hours after her visit that there was a shout: GAS! We all tried to urinate but fear made it impossible. It had to be freshly wet. Some soldiers carried a damp cloth around with them but it was of little use. The gas rolled up our trench. I could smell it long before it reached me but still my rag was dry. We all chided each other: *Come on man, piss for your life!* I did manage a drop but not enough to save my life. The gas got in my throat and up my nose: my lungs were on fire. It made me retch and cough but all that came was blood and then I went blind, my eyes were burning. There were many of us stumbling about, calling for help, but nothing came. Panic ran through the ranks. We were falling about, unable to breathe or see, and then I fell into the mud, others on top of me, too far gone for any help now...

Then Mary was kneeling beside me, holding my head in her little hands, brushing my eyelids with her kisses. I had forgotten the pain I had just felt as she stood and gave me her hand.

I was not alone now. There were many of us all huddled together, holding hands, forming a long line. Then we were flying away from all the sorrow and fear of a war I had not fired a shot in.

I passed from the war to a heavenly place of peace and love, Mary leading the way. She whispered in my ear: *I have a surprise awaiting for you.* Then she showed me two people. I did not have to be told who they were as I knew: Mother and Father. O yes: I was like him, another Barley Boy.

God Bless and thank you for helping to put those fears of dying in tragic conditions behind me; for helping my soul to be free. I've heard say that many a soldier cannot rest in peace till someone like you helps to smooth the way.

Dick (Barley Boy)

Dick passed on 23rd October 1915.

Received on the anniversary of his passing, 23rd October 2008.

I Forsaw My Death in a Dream

I foresaw my death in a troubled dream. I snatched a few moments while there was a lull between fighting on the evening of 17th February 1916. As I sat huddled with my heavy coat around my shoulders, trying to keep warm and dry, I dozed off briefly.

In front of me lay all my comrades fighting had been very heavy with huge loss of life. One by one my mates and close friends fell before me. I saw myself blown to bits. All this flashed through my dream. One moment I was there, the next, no sign of me. I woke with a start: it was only a dream. I had to face so much blood and sorrow since I had been out here no wonder some of the horrors of war infiltrated my dreams.

My name was Alfred, aged 18, from London. Unknown to my fellow mates, I had been psychic from birth and had had many premonitions that came true. I never said what I saw for fear of causing panic among the ranks, but this dream haunted my waking hours.

The damp. Cold morning of the 18th February came. Frozen hands held hot tin mugs of sweet tea, trying to hold a crust of bread. I was hungry: it was our first meal of the day. It was still dark, about an hour to go before the whistle blew. Then, the routine of the day: rifle cleaned and bayonet fixed in place. We all did this without thinking really. It had been drummed into us how our rifle was our best friend. Thoughts whizzed through my mind: what's the use of all this? As this was to be my last day on earth, I sent a message to mam that I would die today and not to grieve too much for me as I would see her again soon. We often communicated this way.

I don't know if this knowledge was an advantage or not. I did not die alone this day. I took with me Matthew from the east end of London and James from Surrey, both 18. Further up the trench was Nigel and Frederick, both 19 and from London. It was a very fierce encounter and I had the task of bugle player, always advance; never retreat. Flack and shell blast and I was gone.

I came today, the 11th November 2008, Remembrance Sunday, when I saw the flame of the candle. Thank you. The names I will give you now all passed with me: Phillip; Andrew; Peter from Sidney, Australia; Ralph from New Zealand; Arthur; Frank; John; Malcolm; so many perished on the Western Front; Corporal Thomas, the Irish Guards; Corporal Phillip, the Somme; Hans, German; Fritz, German; Corporal James; Thomas; Desmond; Dennis, all the Western Front; David, airforce, Lancaster bomber; Jack, ANZAC; Hamish; Jock; Sean; Shaun; Ronald; Sam; Paul; Steven; Michael; Ray; Daniel; Brian; Jess, all 1916, Passchendale; the Somme, Luke, Spitfire.

These are a few of the names given to me on Remembrance Day. I expect that some might come and give me their story later. It was overwhelming being contacted like this, never so many before.

God bless you and thank you for allowing us to talk to you and the peace you have given to me since I passed.

Alfred, aged 18.

Belgian School Master

Hallo. I am Monsieur Michel, a school teacher from a small town on the Belgium/Dutch border. In my school of one class, the children are aged from seven years to fifteen.

After the first attack, our small school was destroyed and I moved all the children into an old farmhouse where I had been born. I felt it was safer there for them. Knowing every inch of the farmhouse, I also knew of the deep cellars and tunnels where I used to play as a child. It was quite dry in there. We stored root vegetables and apples and wine for the winter months. The farm was no longer working as all the young men were enlisted into the German army. I was too old at forty to join up.

But I ran a smooth underground movement to help allied forces to get home as many were left behind. Somehow, the school and the underground worked well together. The Germans were used to seeing me go back and fro with school affairs so took little heed of me. I had two trustworthy friends who I could rely on. We had all been children together. They were the village priest and the local butcher. Their dislike for the Germans was as strong as mine. Our password was *A Baby is Born* meaning that I had someone in hiding.

I successfully moved twenty eight men back to their units or back to England during the first few years of the first world war until my untimely death. It happened when the Germans were moved up to the front line and another unit was moved in. They did not know me or that of my movements with my bike, which the first unit had turned a blind eye to. This lot were of a bad lot. They destroyed our homes and threw out the old folk. They rampaged through our homes and stole our meagre food supplies. We did not like them. I put up with them but mistrusted them all. We Belgians did not like the Germans.

It was later than I thought when I left the farmhouse and cycled back, forgetting the new curfew. A soldier stepped out in front of me and shouted abuse in my face. He would not let me explain why I was out and shot me point blank in the head.

The front line moved back and forward all the time. We got to know the marching of the troops. The British always marched slowly and sang or whistled as they went, but the Germans marched briskly with a strong, hard step and without a word. The locals were out to wave the Tommies on and the children gave them flowers. But the Germans had no welcome from us. In fact, no one was there to see them on their way.

We did not want the war on our doorstep but got caught up in it.

I passed 8th June 1916. Thank you for the chance to at last talk to you, my friend.

Received May 2007

Michel was 5' 7" tall, thin with black hair combed back across his head leaving a high brow. He had brown eyes and wore steel-rimmed glasses. He died aged 46 years old. Time of death: 6.45pm, Sunday 8th June 1916.

Horses of War
First Batallion of Lancers

Strange how we in the spirit world can come to you in thought and you can feel it. Actually, I did come a few nights' ago but you also had others who were in contact with you.

I joined as a cavalry officer. I came over with my own horse. I got a small increase in payment for supplying my own horse. As it turned out, if I had known what was going to happen, I would never have brought Star with me.

It was a very barbaric world I rode into, so different from the quiet countryside of Surrey. I was blind to the thought of what horses had to go through. I wept to see the agony and the ear-splitting screams of the dying horses, their terrified terror scream of pain as they were forced to charge into cannon fire and fences of barbed wire, not the hedges and walls of England's countryside, but blood curdling murder.

On command of charge, swords drawn and held at arms length, we charged into a barrage of cannon fire and a bloody barbed wire fence, too high to jump. What was the use of a sword against bullets? I changed to my hand pistol, like others beside me, but powerless against what we were facing.

The first row of horses fell, followed by row on row, lying in a tangled mess of torn bodies, man and beast all together. My beautiful beast screamed as he was torn to the bone, his velvet brown skin torn to pieces and soaked in his blood. We fell, Star on top of me. I lay there for three days as his blood drained away and his quivering body slowly bled to death.

As the battle raged on and the night came, I heard rifle shots quite close by and German voices as they shot our horses to put them out of their misery and pain. I was so touched with their thoughtfulness. If I had been able, I would have shot him myself. They left us men, especially those who lay under our horses. I was one of those. With the weight of my horse on top of me, I could no longer breath and as the days went on, I got closer to death with each passing hour.

None of us men were told the truth why horses were needed for this barbaric, bloody war. If I had, I would never have put Star through this hell. Slowly I felt my life drain away as I suffocated under horses and men.

Once again I was riding in the green fields of Epsom. Star had no wounds and his velvet skin shone in the early dew. I could not hear his thundering hooves as we flew over fences of beech and hazel, the wind in my hair and all thoughts of war out of my mind. Star and I had been together since I was eighteen years old: now I was twenty-one. My true companion would always be with me.

I was out in Flanders for three weeks only and had ridden into battle twice in that time, coming out unhurt. I blame the ego of the officer who led us out that day as it was a bloody pointless advance. One hundred horses died that day, and as many men, in a fight we never won. Swords against bullets: what utter madness.

My point of view would have been to never involve horses in this kind of pointless war. Horses have been used for generations in warfare, from war in times of knights in full armour, spears, rifles and bows and arrows, centuries of wars, but this was a pointless war to use our beloved animals for.

My name is Hugh. I lived on the edge of Epsom Downs and my dream form a little boy was to be a jockey. I died in June 1916, aged twenty-one.

Hugh came to me. He had blonde-white hair and very green eyes. He stood about 5' 3" tall. He went on to thank me for the help I had given to him and to Star and told me he is the unseen rider way out in front of the race, winning every race, a free spirit and riding all the time, and life in the spirit world is thousands of times better than during those dark days of the bloody war.

Received May 2009.

This story was received five years before the book *War Horse* was shown as a film on TV in 2013. This actually happened for real.

Canadian Soldier 1916

Here I was, sitting, leaning back against hard wooden slats on the Great Canadian Railway (steam train, green and brass) off to war, leaving my beloved homeland behind me, of rushing rivers, tumbling waterfalls, dark forests of fir. High mountains topped with snow, and mirrored lakes so clear and beautiful. All this was part of the British Empire so when a call was heard, call to arms, you are needed to fight and defend the British Empire against the Germans who were sweeping across Europe like a raging forest fire, we did not hesitate to go.

There were twenty men from my side of Canada, riding the troop train as it made its way following the river, picking up more men on its way. Sitting on these hard seats in new uniforms, so stiff the khaki uniform, it scuffed my neck, rubbed sore under my arms, in my groin and behind my knees. The boots were not a comfortable fit but we were told they would break in when we were marching.

Gazing out of the steamed up carriage window, this was my first trip I had ever taken on a train, so seeing the countryside rush by I let my mind wander. I was a child again, running beside the train, swimming rivers, climbing mountains…

All too soon the vistas of Canada as I remember it were melting away, and tall buildings and factory chimneys came in view and talk of Seattle was heard. This was where we'd embark onto a troop ship and sail to Britain. With a sinking feeling, I knew I would never come home again. Monty was my eldest brother, by two years. He had joined up to join the Flying Corps. We had news just before I left that he was missing in action and Mother's parting words were *Find Monty.*

I was proud to wear the King's uniform. My name was Bart, short for Bartholomew, aged eighteen, and Monty was short for Montgomery, aged twenty. I carried a creased photo of him standing beside his Tiger Moth plane taken somewhere in England. He lived for flying. Every day I would hold his photo and talk to him. I joined the army. I was no longer a farmer's son, a green horn, but a young man going to war so far from home.

I was brought sharply back to the present time: shouts; orders; marching in time. We moved as one long line to board the ship that would take us to England.

The sea journey was anything but safe with a huge fleet of German subs hunting us and tracking our every move. We came under fire but we sunk the sub with our torpedoes. I was dreadfully sea sick and was glad to land safely after many weeks at sea.

I was tall and lean with brown hair and dark hazel eyes and a square jaw, looking like my father. Monty was about as tall as myself but was blond and looked like my mother. He was a very bright boy who did well in anything he did. I, on the other hand, was slower to act, always the little brother, with few guts to try anything new.

But I was good at following orders and father had said that the army life would make a man out of me. Monty's letters home were few but the ones we got, mother would re read them, placing the letter against her heart with tears in her eyes. I wondered if they would do the same with mine.

When I came over, I forgot to mention that the troop ship also carried doctors, nurses, replacement weapons and horses. I spent many a long hour below deck tending the horses. They gave me great comfort but I am sure I helped them in their dark, unnatural quarters. I felt sure that they also felt sick like us landlubbers.

Embarkation was at Southampton. We were changed to a different troop ship to cross the English Channel. We could not go right up to the shore to land but were transferred onto a landing craft which took us up onto the beach. The horses were the last to go ashore.

The Canadian fall was in its glory when I left home: now it was a cold, late December day, bleak and very raw, damp. I was not used to weather like this. My boots hurt: we all suffered from raw rubbed heels and toes but were told that walking would harden our lily-white feet and by the time we reached the front line, the rain would mould the boots to our feet. It was just a case of grin and bear it, as our British soldier mates told us.

Then, in ranks, we started to march. The constant drumming of hundreds of feet carried us forward into a land so strange and so far from home, with rifles against our right shoulder, a kit bag so heavy that it hung low and bumped our backs. We marched all day, only stopping for a drink of water in a small village along the way where a few small children handed us little bunches of wild flowers and waved us forward.

By nightfall we rested in a barn. It had been used before as I found an English wrapper from some kind of food tin. Glad for a moment to unburden my weary back and eat food was a welcome change to a long day's marching but sleep did not come peacefully to me as I could hear the rumble of cannon fire somewhere up ahead. But finally sleep hung heavy on my eyelids as I dozed into an uneasy sleep.

Daybreak came so fast. A meal was eaten and hot, sweet tea brought me awake to another day closer to where we were heading. The morning heralded a cold, pale, winter sun but at least it was dry, to start with. Rain hit us by midday and never stopped long enough for us to dry out again.

All day we could hear the rumble of guns, getting louder by the mile. Surely the war would end soon. It had been two years of fighting, it must be nearly over by now. Then we saw mile on mile of rough, wooden crosses all along the road side with some scribbled names on them. Dog tags were of little use to mark a grave as they were either made of card, only officers had wooden ones: that's why so many soldiers have never been found. My dog tag, as it was named, was about two inches long with my rank number and name on one side and on the other my regiment and the red maple leaf. It looked very smart when it was first put around my neck but even now it was starting to wear at the edges.

There was a sweet smell. Later we learnt it was the dead. By the time we reached the mud-soaked trenches, the smell of death was so strong that it filled our nostrils like a heavy cold which we could not get rid of. The dead lay where they fell. There was no time to come back to bury our dead. Word got round about the wooden crosses. They were graves dug by the villagers as the fighting moved up the line to new defence positions but the death count grew daily. Thousands had already died in this foreign land, far from home, and had never had a grave. I asked if anyone had seen Monty, as a pilot, but most said that they had not seen any planes.

Finally we were at a place called Athies: this was our front line. We saw the ruins of a small church high on a hill above the small town. The place was almost deserted.

It was now the end of August 1917, dug in, in mud with flies and the stench of the dead which we had grown used to. Sitting in my own grave although not dead, but buried alive. A machine gun post some few hundred feet from my right had us pinned down for days, unable to move forward or to blast it off the face of the earth. Machine gun bullets whizzed past my ear. I could actually feel the whip of air as it went past. Which bullet would have my name on it? A fraction to the left and I would be dead. I had time to talk to Monty. I felt sure he must be dead as I had not found out anything about him for nearly ten months.

We edged forward inch by inch. We were heavily outnumbered by the German military force of the equipment: guns and ammo; tanks; and men who never seemed to get less like we did. In the early hours of the dawn I heard my name being called: *Bart, be careful.* Taken by utter surprise, I stood up and was shot through the head. Boy oh boy: is that what it feels like to be shot? Then Monty was beside me, laughing. *I tried to warn you, little brother, but I did not think that you would be so stupid to actually stand up!*

Hand in hand, Monty and I walked away from the battlefield, reunited again. It was on the third day of September 1917.

Talking to you made me realize that there is life after death. Thank you.

The Son of my Father – Cuthbert's Story

Good day, Lady. I was the first son, born into the gentry. Father was a retired cavalry officer from Balaclava and it was expected that I should follow father into the army. I had no choice. I was told that this is your destiny, my man. Army and battles were shown in large black oil paintings which covered the walls of my home, each showing one relation or other through the years, in massive grounds in Wiltshire.

At the age of seventeen I had been groomed to be a soldier. At the tender age of make believe, of climbing trees or just playing as small children do, I would be called to my father's study to play war games. Father would never allow me to be a little boy. I dreaded these hours of war games and tactics. I would obediently sit at his feet to go through another battle campaign.

At seventeen, I took a commission, missing all the lower ranks and coming out as a captain in the cavalry.

My name was Cuthbert. I grew up hardly ever seeing Mama, just a goodnight kiss and the sweet smell of rose water on her cheeks. My early days of life had been in a nursery. I can see it now, plainly, as I lie in a dug-out in the blistering heat and flies of Palestine in 1917.

I was in the cavalry, not with horses but with camels. Quite a different animal to ride – smelly, bad-tempered and headstrong, foaming at the mouth and spitting. I often would smile just to think what father would have said. At first we all felt sea-sick, riding this ship of the desert, but strangely enough it was quite comfortable.

I had been in Palestine for three months when I was shot. The Padre came and gave me communion and to pray with me. I found his words comforting but I knew that I would never set foot on home land again. My wounds were fatal. As I lay, my batman waved the flies off my face and wet my lips with cool water but I was not fully conscious of what was going on around me. I took a long time to die. I had been shot in the back and could not feel my legs. I felt no pain. When my time at last came, I knew that the next generation would never have stories of war thrust down their throats of the glories of battle. It was not the glory of dying as in fact my father never was wounded or actually knew what it was like to die.

Now I was with my Bessie. She was my nanny and I loved her dearly. Those warm, winter afternoons in my nursery, playing childhood games, riding my rocking horse, Dobbin, tea beside a cheery fire and stories of King Arthur. No war games but just a little boy with love and hugs from Bessie. I never really knew my mother.

Now if only father could see me: a reluctant soldier who didn't want to go to war, dying in the hot sands of Palestine so far away from home on 11th August 1917.

Cuthbert describes himself as tall with blond, unruly hair and blue eyes. He had a gentle face and no strong chin or jawline like his father. He tells me he was scared of his bullying father and that's why he took all the lessons he was taught and never argued with him. Cuthbert was just eighteen when he died.

Received January 2007

The Good Shepherd

Thousands of years ago, a story was told starting with Christ as The Good Shepherd.

A shepherd in Palestine knew every sheep he had, and if one went missing or astray, he would search until he found and returned it to the fold. A fold was usually a low stone wall made of whatever was at hand. Branches were often used so to confine his sheep and he would lie down across the entrance to guard his flock from wolves. He did not have a dog. He would lead his sheep by walking in front of them: where he went, they followed.

There is another true story handed down from father to son for generations, from one shepherd to another.

In Yorkshire and Cumbria, it was a known fact that when a shepherd died and his body laid to rest, a piece of fleece was wound around his fingers to show St. Peter he was a shepherd and could not find time to go to church, as was expected of him. St. Peter would see that this man was a good shepherd and would let him pass.

I would like to know whether this old custom is still practised.

I found this story amongst my late father's sermons which were written over sixty years ago.

The Shepherd

I had a dream that I was on the hills on my remote sheep farm in Wales near the Black Mountains. It was my father's farm but my responsibility was the care of the sheep. I was a shepherd.

I am Gweyn Hughes, twenty four years of age, a big man in stature with black, curly hair, grey eyes and large gentle hands. I could drive in a fence post with my fist yet on the other hand, gentle enough to help bring a little lamb into the world. I had three brothers older than myself and one sister, younger. That's why I am here now. In my dream I was sitting on the hillside helping with the ewes at the time of lambing. It was a cold night and the black, moonless sky was peppered with twinkling stars. Sitting, leaning against my leg, Lass, my favourite collie dog. I often did the night watch in March at lambing time. Hearing the first small bleat of new life: oh, such happy times! I'd do anything to be there again.

Coming out of my dream, I still felt something warm leaning against my leg. Looking down, I saw a wounded soldier leaning against me for support in the muddy trench on a cold May night in 1917.

A May night would be full of nightingale song and fire flies back home. Apple blossom, bluebells and bird song would herald a new day. But I knew today was going to be my last day on earth. It was dark with a fine drizzle, the damping kind that would soak you to the skin, one that would never dry out. Since being out here for one and a half months, I had only seen the sun twice: not a warming sun but a watery one, showing a pale glimmer in a foggy sky.

Thinking of my family, I stood up on command to go over the top when the whistle blew. Somehow I knew that one of those bullets would have my name on it.

We had been under heavy bombardment from enemy lines for hours. You could hear the bullets whiz past your ears: not that one but maybe the next. We came close to dying every hour of every day but that bullet did not have my name on it. We talked about how we would die. All of us without exception said that a bullet to the head was the best way to go, you would not feel a thing. Young men were being sick. They threw up all around me, faces grey with anguish and fear, shaking and praying to come back alive. But I felt calm. I was not going to give way to emotions. I had faced fear many times in my life.

The shrill blast of the whistle brought me back from my wandering thoughts of home and I was climbing up the ladder to go over the top as I had done so many times before. The flimsy ladder barely carried my weight. I was left handed so would carry my rifle in the wrong hand. Officers would keep telling me to change hands but it was useless: I could only do it my way. Stooping low, I started to run forward with the others. My pals were dropping like flies beside me. Then a bullet with my name on it went straight through my helmet: I never felt a thing. It was true that I did not know that I was dead: it happened so fast.

Gathering up my fellow comrades, we walked back to our trench, unseen by all the others. Our war was over.

It took me a long time to come to terms with my death. Finally talking to you last night, in your dreams, I can now move on and forward to the light and live in peace.

Thank you, my new friend, for helping me over.

Gweyn Hughes. May 1917.

Received 7th December 2006

Harry, War Animals, 1917

Hallo. I am Harry. I joined up with all the other boys in my village and enlisted and was over in Belgium before they realised I was too young to fight. I got jostled along with the idea that this would be an adventure, given the King's Shilling, the first coin I had ever held.

When they found out I was only fifteen, I was given the job of looking after the pigeons, feeding them and fastening little messages to their tiny legs. These brave little birds would fly criss-cross over the battle fields relaying messages. Often, they were shot down and eaten, though a few always got through.

I lived for the animals. It was not only the pigeons that I cared for. There were the dogs. Some had come with their masters and most were used to carry packs of first aid or metal containers with bullets and cartridges to gun positions. Others were used to search out the living from the dead in No Man's Land when it was dark and fighting had stopped for the night.

My favourite little dog was called Titch. He was a small terrier who would go off on his own, always knowing who needed a warm lick on his face, to comfort the tired and frightened men. He would sit on their lap and snuggle up for a hug. Often, it was said, many would hide their faces in his fur and cry. He often came back thick with mud but he always had time for anyone who needed help and comfort.

Horses broke my heart. How could Man treat these noble creatures like this? Many were someone's pet. When the people of England were asked to give a horse to help with the war, no one ever thought that their race horse or child's pet would ever live like this. They would never see them again, although they were promised by the military that they would come back. Gentle creatures, shaking with shell shock; ears flat on their heads; whites of eyes rolling in fear. The stable boy would tell me dreadful stories, of which I'm telling you a bit. And their screams of terror would haunt me.

I died in a mustard attack while waiting for the birds to come back. They started to fall out of the sky, their feathers yellow with dust, choking, little birds unable to breath. I was meant to be safe, well behind the lines, but it depended on the direction of the wind and how strong it was. The Germans were the first to use it. Sometimes the wind would change and they got it back. I did not have time to run back for the mask. I could not see. I was choking, my lungs fit to burst. I died in agony before any help came. The last thing I remember was waiting for my birds to come back and seeing them drop out of the sky like a little yellow ball of feathers.

The sergeant was very kind to me. He called me "son" as I cried a lot and he handed me a tin mug of sweet, hot tea. I would wrap my frozen fingers around the mug and sip the hot liquid that had a very faint taste of tea, not like mum's tea. I left this earth on 3rd September, two days after my sixteenth birthday.

Received 17th October 2009.

Coal Mining Engineer Gilbert's Story

Hallo, I am Gilbert, aged 45 years old and I lived in Wales. A call went out for mining engineers to dig and construct a bunker underground. The ordinary soldier didn't have the knowledge: we coal miners had. The offer of better wages than we were getting made it sound interesting. They, The War Office, wanted men with experience, the older the better, so, leaving my wife, Blodwyn and four children, I headed for the front lines in 1917.

The large, underground bunker had to be at least ninety feet deep, with wooden sides and corrugated iron roofing. It was a big task. I was put in charge of the men. They were mainly young miners ranging in age from 18 to 40. I was the oldest.

This bunker was to have an officers' room and bunk areas for ranks of importance. The other soldiers, the young men on the front lines, did not have the luxury of sleeping in the dry. We worked in tunnels of damp earth. Our only light was that of a solitary candle. At least we did not inhale coal dust. And with the candle there was no fear of a gas explosion. Timbers were cut above ground to my specifications, no bolts were used, but one piece of timber would slot into another. It was real art.

We earned the nickname of "Vampyres" as we seldom saw the light of day. We had eight hours down and six hours up when we would fill sandbags for the shoring up of the sides of the trenches as we needed to get rid of all the earth we dug out. We were fed and then returned down to sleep till it was time to start all over again. When it was possible, the injured were brought down as temporary shelter till there was a lull in the fighting or when it became dark: then stretcher bearers came and the wounded were taken away.

Sometimes we could feel the sudden vibration of shell blast as we were digging well below No Man's Land and my heart and prayers went out to our young men who were shedding their blood above us.

I came from a small village outside Bangor. My time on earth ended on 17th September 1917 when there was a cave-in, when hundreds of tons of mud and water fell on me, crushing me to death: no one could save me. Although most of the soil was heavy with clay, it could also be water-logged, making the digging heavy-going at the best of times.

As it was, the job we undertook to do for the army never really came to an end. There was always other tunnels and bunkers to dig. We were promised that when this bunker was done, we would be sent home, but that never happened. I left a lovely family behind and was looking forward to having my first two grandchildren.

Thank you for your attention and care for taking down my story. There would never be a "Welcome in the Hillsides" for me again.

Received on 5th November 2008, several weeks before the BBC programme telling us about the Vampyre Bunker of WWI. But this is evidence that this contact with soldiers is correct at the time I received it.

Spotter Plane

I flew a bi-plane during the Battle of the Somme in 1917 my job was to fly over enemy front lines and report back their positions while taking photographs of the situation. What our side wanted to know was what strength the troops were and how many tanks and machine guns there were.

I only had six hours flying time. They needed a volunteer and I stepped forward: anything to be able to fight! I had seen no action yet.

A heavy camera with big plates for the photographs was fitted to the right side of my plane. This was a single-handed operation. Later, the plane would have two men to operate the camera and to fly the plane.

I had to fly over their front lines, directly in front of their guns. It was a case of flying out of the sun, if the sun was out, swoop low, take the photograph, change the plate of glass being careful not to drop it, then replace it and do it again. The Germans used to use me as a target and blast off their guns. When I got my picture, I would rise sharply, do a roll and head back to my side of the the front lines. I got to know the German spotter pilot. As we raced across, passing each other, we started to salute each other. It was like a game of cat and mouse.

I never really took this job as seriously as I should have. It was like a game as I loved flying. The sensation of flying like a bird in effortless flight, free, with a bird's eye view of tiny people far below. I was never in all that war, fighting and bloodshed. I had to make the most of my freedom while it lasted as one never knew how long we had.

Looking down on fields and tiny houses, and yet unspoilt woods from where I sat in my little plane made from paper and string. I never knew what kept it up so long. I heard no sound of gun fire or blast of cannon fire, no smell of death or screams from man or beast.

Until all that changed when I swooped down for my final pass and some black movement caught my eye. I put my plane into a nose dive to take the one and last picture, pulling up as I swept over the front lines. I had done this manoeuvre many times but this time my plane would not pull up. Glancing wildly around me, I saw oil coming from the fuselage, then smoke and flames: all this in a split moment as I hurtled to my death. There was no time to jump but then the fall would also have killed me.

The Air Vice Marshall who gave us training said that it was not practical to give us anything to help us escape. It was a case of going down with your plane, the sacrifice we had to bear. But the Germans had a type of wing thing to jump and float down, but we did not. It would later be called a parachute and used in the next wars but in this war we had nothing to save our lives. My life ended long before I hit the ground, by a loud explosion and a ball of flames as my flimsy plane burst into flame as the engine plummeted to the ground.

When I first joined up, I had a young lad with me. His name was Harry. He was too young to fight at fifteen so got the job of looking after the animals. You might hear from him

Antony was a plump lad of eighteen years old, with freckles and red hair and grey eyes. He says it was a joke with the flying group as his commander said he would never fit into the cockpit as he was too fat. But I turned out to be one of the best fliers of my time. He tells me that as a child he would make little planes out of wood, tied together with whatever he could find, throwing them into the air in his back garden which had little room for a child to play in as it was stacked high with junk. His father was a rag and bone man and it was his destiny to follow in his father's trade but ever since he saw his first plane, all he wanted was to fly like a bird.

Antony passed in July 1917 in a place called Athies.

Received January 2008.

47

HMS Dreadnought 1906 – 1922

Hallo, I'm Frank, the oldest of a large brood of children, born in Plymouth in 1891. at the age of fourteen I was employed as an apprentice in Portsmouth shipyards as a very junior shipwright. I don't know why at the time but we had a rushed job to build this large battleship, the most powerful girl ever to be built in my lifetime. She was to be called HMS Dreadnought, an 18110 ton battleship built at Portsmouth dockyard. She represented one of the most notable design steam turbine power plant and at 21 knot maximum speed, she was the best and over powered all the previous ones as "pre-dreadnoughts."

The swiftness of her construction was incredible. We laid down the foundations in October 1905 and she was launched in February 1906 after only four months.

The Dreadnought was closely watched by the US Navy's Officer of Naval Intelligence and the world's naval authorities. Dreadnought first served as the flag ship of the Home Fleet from 1907 to 1922.

After she was launched, I enrolled to be on board to serve with her. She was the first battleship I had the honour to build. The crew of the Dreadnought was made up mostly of the men who had built her. It numbered five hundred men: welders; carpenters; designers, and engineers. Once the keel was laid, she was a magnificent queen of the seas. No one in the world had finer ship builders than the British as a nation of seafarers. I always wondered how such a ship could float.

I joined the navy as I felt I wanted to learn more than just building ships when I had the chance. There were whispers of war. What if? I served with the 4th Battle Squadron in the North Sea during the First World War. During the first two years of the war, on 18th March 1915, we rammed and sank the German submarine U29. We spent days searching out German subs: this is what she was built to do. I never for one moment thought she would ever be hit or sunk. She was our little bit of England, firm and strong, and we all loved her dearly.

Dreadnought was always the flagship. She was built with booms from her sides to support anti-torpedo nets. Her anchor was suspended from her starboard deck when under way.

After target practice, King Edward VII visited in July 1907, she flew the Royal Standard at her foremast, mid ships and her target mast at her stern.

We served in the Mediterranean in 1906. Guns were added with shields for her twelve powder guns and her main mast had been removed.

I saw a lot of the world and a lot of action as well.

I don't suppose a lot of this information I have given you makes a lot of sense but anyone who has served in the navy would expect the correct details of this very fine British battleship to be correct.

As I have mentioned, I was 22 years old at the beginning of the first world war.

I left the navy when, in 1922, the Dreadnought left active duty and was based at the Thames to counter the threat of bombardment by German battle cruisers and was placed in reserve in 1919. I followed her life and fond memories of being actually there when she was born. So, in 1922 she was sold for scrap. With foresight I don't think Britain ever thought there would be another war but by then she would have been out of date. A big part of me died with her.

Back home again after the war, I found that my family had suffered great losses with the deaths of two of my brothers. Jack and Steven had joined up in the army and had died in Flanders trenches. Tom returned home suffering from shell shock and was blind. Like thousands of other men we came home to a devastated and very poor country, and finding work of any kind was impossible, with thirty men seeking the same job, those of us who could work.

I was lucky to find a little work with a roof over my head. Mother could not cope with Tom, it was too much for her so I took Tom and looked after him till his death a few months later aged 20. I joined the fire brigade and enjoyed the work and the thrill of danger. I felt at home with an organised life of rules, like my navy days.

I was too old to join up again when the second world war broke so stayed with the fire service. I was 48 years old in 1939 when my life came to a sudden end. It happened one stormy night while we were fighting a huge warehouse fire down on the docks after a bombing raid. With strong winds fanning up mountains of flames, one wall of the warehouse toppled over, crushing me. It was days before they found me. It was in 1939.

Thank you for taking time to write all this down: just another lost soul found and given rest. I was met by my comrades and my two brothers. There were so many to welcome me home.

Received October 2008

Henry

Hallo, it's nice to meet up with you at long last. I have heard about the kind people who help us tormented souls find peace and your name was spoken of more than anyone else. So I hope you don't mind me making contact with you. I am Henry, aged 22, born in Winchester in 1918.

It is now the summer of 1940 and I'm flying a Spitfire. If you were standing looking up at the vapour trails snaked across the sky, recording the life or death dog fights between the Spits and the Messerschmidts, the fight was known as the Battle for Britain. The fight lasted four months. We were called by Churchill *The Few:* 2936 young pilots took to the air to protect our English soil from Germany's power. They seemed to have so many planes to our few. 544 pilots died, many were lost at sea, never to be found. I was one of the last to be killed. Some said I had a charmed life as I had so many hours flying time and my kills numbered 12, quite good really. You had to report how many you had shot down.

My time came one hot, summer's afternoon. I started the day with Lucy crowding my thoughts. I don't know why as you could not afford to be distracted for one moment. Sitting in my cockpit, twisting my neck back and forth to see if there was enemy aircraft near: nothing in sight, when Leader One called out a warning that I had Jerry on my tail. Bullets whizzed through my fuselage and I lost control of my plane. Then I was in flames, hurtling towards the sea.

The next thing I remember was sitting on the playing fields watching my school play cricket.

My life as a pilot, in those far off days of war, was firing at the enemy, going to refuel and up again. Those days of excitement kept us going.

Thank you for the healing to help me: God bless you.

I lost my best buddy on the same day as I died. His name was Cyril. I know he is waiting to follow me. He was 5' 9" tall. of slim build with blond hair and hazel eyes. He tells me he always stood up for the underdog.

Received 5/4/08

Dogfight for the Battle of Britain

Hallo, friend. My mate has just been been in contact with you. We were great buddies, joining up the same day, doing our training and then going into the war together. Henry was a top pilot and lived a charmed life with many brushes with death but he always came back to base. Better tell you something about me. My name was Cyril, nickname Cy. I am 20 years old with little or no education as I ran away from school more than I was ever in class. I came from a broken home where my mother could not control me.

My home was in Kent. Then I got interested in planes, and at the age of 14 all I wanted was to fly. I met Henry who helped me to read and to pass my flying exams. We were inseparable after that. The main target of the air force was to take public school boys and make them into officers but so many were killed that they were desperate for more pilots. That's how I now flew a Spitfire.

By the time I was ready to fly, the Battle for Britain had been fighting for three months.

I had just started to take notice of the real danger I was in. flying high in the beautiful blue summer sky of a really hot summer of 1940 when my final day came, I saw Henry dive into the sea. I was so afraid for him that I broke ranks and tried to follow him down to see if he was still alive. The sky was full of Messerschmitts and also the heavy bombers of the Luftwaffe coming in for a bombing raid on London.

I got hit by friendly fire as the ack-ack guns blasted off at the bombers. I got caught in the cross fire. When pilots fly into the sun, a shadow across your view, you are blinded for a split second. I don't blame anyone – it was entirely my own fault as I was in the wrong place at that moment of time.

I felt so calm, looking about me. My bullet-proof windscreen was shot away. The force of the cold air crushed my lungs and I was plummeting into the sea. I did not have time to use my parachute.

Henry and I met up, and once again I felt safe that he was with me.

Thank you for your help. Just talking to you has filled the empty pages of my life and has filled them with hope.

Cy was of a stocky build with a mass of black hair and had brown eyes. He had not started to shave yet.

Received 5/4/08

My Hurricane

At last, I've made contact with you. My name was Timothy. I was twenty-one when I left this earth in 1940, September the twelfth.

I was stationed at RAF Hawking in Kent, only a few miles from where I lived with my parents. I flew a Hurricane, trained and got my wings to fly six months after the outbreak of war. Here we all were, ready and very eager to shoot down the enemy before they got us.

The battle we were fighting was a great air battle over the sea and the south coast of England. It would be known as the Battle of Britain. Our small group of Spitfires and Hurricanes were grossly outnumbered by the German Luftwaffe and Messerschmitts. This battle took place from August to October 1940, one continuous fight from dawn to dusk. We never thiught that you would be shot down. We were far superior fliers than the Germans. We flew rings round them. Every available pilot was called up.

1940 was a hot summer. The dawns came in bright, the skies were blue and the evenings lingered for a long time. Winston Churchill called us "The Few": true, we were but a few but we fought like a full squadron, shoulder to shoulder.

I am afraid I never saw the end of our dog fights namely called because we hunted our prey down, round and round, flying throttle full out, diving, rise roll: it was exciting, boys with toys my mother said we were.

Flying became my life in those short months of the war. Once I left the ground, I became a bird, the wings of my plane became my wings: I was flying. Our main target was to protect our beautiful island from invasion. Then I was falling. I had no control of my wings. A shot bird, I plummeted to the earth. I did not live to hit the ground but the next thing I knew, I was standing beside my plane, a burnt out wreckage, in a cool wood in a clearing that my plane had made by crashing through the canopy of trees.

I had no pain, I was not burnt. A great flow of peace and quiet surrounded me. It was then I saw a little girl of about six years old. We stood and stared at each other. She was not afraid but said: *I will go and get Daddy. He will know what to do.*

I was traumatised at the sudden way I had died and kept going back to my plane until one day I just gave up as no one had come for me. I did not know that I was dead: I knew that I was lost. Then someone said: *Go to Margaret, she will help you.* So, here I am. Thank you for your prayers and for making me better. I can now move on.

Received September 2004.

HMS Hood

Good day, lady. My name is Alfie. I was a sailor: in fact, I was chief stoker aboard HMS Hood during the second world war. Hood was a massive iron battleship. I used to marvel how it could float, but she did.

We were returning from a trip in the north Atlantic in May 1941. We were travelling in a convoy so we thought we were safe. We developed engine trouble and were left behind. It was not noticed that we were no longer in the convoy. We had to have radio silence as the Atlantic was very well covered by the German navy. When we disappeared off the radar it was too late: we were at the bottom of the sea.

We had picked up the battleship the Bismark. She was just out of range of our guns but moving slower. They attacked us with all their heavy guns and the next thing I knew a shell blast hit our ammunition room, exploding, which sunk us.

But before this happened, we had just received a message to say that the east end of London had been badly bombed that night. I lived there with my wife, Mabel, aged 23, and my two little ones,

Alfred, 3 years old, and Jane, just 1 year old. All were killed. I was devastated by the news we were going home to nothing but sorrow.

My job was stoker. Once the engine trouble had been fixed and we were able to get up steam, the protecting convoy was nowhere to be seen, and if they had turned around to come back for us, it was too late. The Bismark had been hunting us all day but our guns were not made for long range firing. We sank. 1415 hands were lost; only 3 lives were saved.

Being down below, I was unaware of the situation on deck. The conditions were hot and dusty and I would rush up on occasions to grab a lungful of fresh air before going down again. With steam up to power, I was waiting for word from the bridge to change course but it never came.

When death stares you in the face, there is nothing you can do. Your life, once so strong and living, is now fragile, like a candle flame in a strong wind, easily blown out.

The Hood sank very fast: no time to launch lifeboats. Panic swallowed us as the sea rushed in. the explosion blew me to bits. Being below, I had no idea of the desperate situation on deck and the next thing I knew was my last thought on this earth.

I had joined the navy in the 1900s and having been well-educated, I had a love of words. When my fellow mates heard about this, I often wrote love letters to their families and loved ones.

Thank you for helping me to face my life and to remove the fear of the terrifying memories that have haunted me for so long. At the moment of my death, all my family was with me.

Alfie.

Received 5th August 2007.

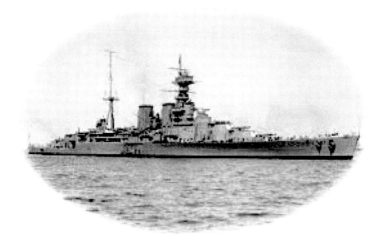

Bismark

When news reached England that HMS Hood had been sunk in May 1941, Winston Churchill ordered the sinking of the Bismark as a priority to the safety of the Merchant Navy and all British ships. Within three days the Bismark was sunk with the loss of all hands. 2,200 were drowned. She sank with all her flags flying.

My name is Fritz. I am 21 years old, a gunner on board of our most powerful German navy. It was I who fired the fatal shell that sunk the Hood and I would get the Iron Cross for my bravery. I was so proud of what I had done. We all celebrated that evening.

The Bismark had been following the Hood, keeping just outside the reach of her guns until our chance came, when the Hood slowed down and her convoy of merchant ships seemed to leave her behind. This was the chance we had been waiting for. We were no longer in any danger from her escort ships. The Bismark's main task was to hunt down the British navy and sink them all. We were a superior race to the British. We outnumbered them three to one. We had been told that the German forces were the best in the world: at sea; in the air, and on land. Everyone must fight for the Fatherland, so we did.

We got the reputation of being the wolf pack, hunting down all British ships, and so far we had done an excellent job. But our glory days were coming to an end. For all her strength, the Bismark did not stand a chance against the whole British navy. They all turned on us, hunting us from below the waves to the surface ships. We just were run down. I had no idea how many ships the British actually had. We had been led to believe that we were the most powerful navy afloat. We were also sought by air. A torpedo from a plane sunk us. After the British sunk us, they continued to hunt us from the air and sea.

As a gunner, we took no prisoners. I would shoot all survivors: their calls for help went unheeded. I just hated them all. I still could hear the words, that we were a superior race and we must not let our feelings crowd out the need to win every fight. So this is how I was.

But now I was in the water. How cold it was. The power of the sea and the force of the ship going down pulled me under. I could not get free. So this is what it felt like, being helpless, in icy waters with no one to come and rescue me.

With the tragic loss of our greatest ship, it was the start of us losing the war. Germany's heart died.

I was six feet tall with blond hair and blue eyes. In my youth, I was one of Hitler's Youth Army before joining the navy. I was Lutheran: well, it did me no good. I am here now. It took me a long time to stop hating my enemy. My enemy is just like me: there is no difference with skin colour, we now all look the same. It did not help me moving forward while I had so much hate in my heart.

Thank you for hearing my side of the war. I was surprised when I made contact with you, that you accepted me for what I am.

Fritz

Received March 2009

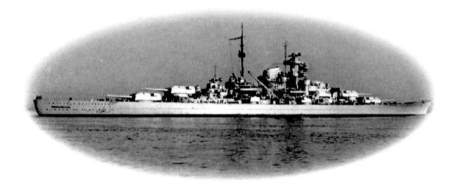

Poem

"Please wear a poppy," the lady said
And held one forth, but I shook my head.
Then I stopped and watched as she offered them there,
And her face was old and lined with care;
But beneath the scars the years had made
There remained a smile that refused to fade.

A boy came whistling down the street,
Bouncing along on care-free feet.
His smile was full of joy and fun,
"Lady," said he, "may I have one?"
When she'd pinned one on he turned to say,
"Why do we wear a poppy today?"

The lady smiled in her wistful way
And answered, "This is Remembrance Day,
And the poppy there is the symbol for
The gallant men who died in the war.
And because they did, you and I are free –
That's why we wear a poppy, you see.

"I had a boy about your size,
With golden hair and big blue eyes.
He loved to play and jump and shout,
Free as a bird he would race about.
As the years went by he learned and grew
and became a man – as you will too.

"He was fine and strong, with a boyish smile,
But he'd seemed with us such a little while
When war broke out he went away.
I still remember his face that day
When he smiled at me and said, "Goodbye,
I'll be back soon, Mom, so please don't cry."

"But the war went on and he had to stay,
And all I could do was wait and pray.
His letters told of the awful fight,
(I can see it still in my dreams at night),
With the tanks and guns and cruel barbed wire,
And the mines and bullets, the bombs and fire.

"Till, at last, the war was won –
And that's why we wear a poppy, son."
The small boy turned as if to go,
Then said, "Thanks, lady, I'm glad to know.
That sure did sound like an awful fight,
But your son – did he come back all right?"

A tear rolled down each faded cheek;
She shook her head, but didn't speak.
I slunk away in a sort of shame,
And if you were me you'd have done the same;
For our thanks, in giving, if oft delayed,
Thought our freedom was bought – and thousands paid!

And so when we see a poppy worn,
Let us reflect on the burden borne,
By those who gave their very allowing
When asked to answer their country's call
That we at home in peace might live.
Then wear a poppy! Remember – and give!

Don Crawford

Hell Fire Pass

I was born in Ceylon in 1904, a son of a tea plantation owner. My father was British and my mother was Ceylonese. He ran his father-in-law's tea plantation but when he died, I took over and at the age of sixteen ran it with my grandfather. It was later sold and I was given my share of the profits, enough to buy myself a tea plantation of my own.

I heard that in the high lands of Burma the land was very fertile and tea grew well. So, leaving the plantation, I thought I would first go back to England to visit my relations and see a bit of the world as I had never left Ceylon. Then back to Burma to look for the tea plantation I had heard about.

Ceylon was part of the British Empire and had a great loss of man power during the first world war. Visiting England at the end of that war was not what I had thought it to be like. Father had always painted such a lush, green land. Mother died when I was 19 in 1922.

Boarding a train at Rangoon, heading north to Mandalay, reaching Burma in the spring of 1932, I sought out the tea plantation that I had been told about. It had been neglected badly and therefore it was a price that suited me well. On closer inspection I noticed that more than three quarters of the tea bushes were dead and had to be pulled out and burned.

I inherited the men and their numerous families who were living in the most appalling conditions. So homes had to be the first target, as a happy worker is a good worker. Plans were drawn out and timber cut and houses built. I gave them six weeks to do this, all hands to work.

My house needed repairing also but that could wait. In the meantime, with one or two of the older men, I started to pull out and burn the dead bushes. Ox and plough had to be used to clear the ground and new tea bushes had to come up from Ceylon to replace my fields: this all took time. So, by late summer, we were ready for the first harvest. I was so happy in my work with all the plans for the future. I had seventeen good and reliable workers, and repairs to my roof were done before the monsoons came.

The years flew by and news drifted through that a second world war was coming. Burma was under attack from the Japs while the Germans were pushing through Europe like wildfire. I did not think that this war would effect me, but I was wrong.

My plantation was set in the area of Manipur. Just across the valley was the start of dense jungle which ran across the Indian border. One day, when out on horseback, I came across the body of a dog hanging by its neck, left to die. This was a barbaric thing done around here. I could not leave it there so I cut it down only to discover that it was still alive. Now what was I going to do? So I lifted it up onto my saddle and took it home.

He was a large, black dog with one white paw. I nursed him back to health and he followed me everywhere. I called him Spark. It was good to have a watch dog as people were coming and going across my land as the panic of war spread. One day, he started to bark, long before I heard anything: army Jeeps were winding their way up the valley to the house. I was sitting on the veranda, sipping green tea, watching the sun dip into the sea hundreds of miles off the horizon: the best time of day to relax after a heavy day in the fields.

In 1939 war had broken out in Europe but still that was nothing to do with me. England was at war with Germany. Then, in 1940, war drums started to beat in the far east as the Japs took hold of Malaysia and Singapore, swarming across to Burma and into India, through Hell Fire Pass, which I would get involved with. I knew it would be any time now so when the army Jeep trundled up our steep road to the house, I was half expecting it.

A tall English major unfolded himself out of the seat, brushing off the dust of the road and striding up the steps. Spark came swiftly to my side to protect me. I stood to meet him. He introduced himself , shaking me by the hand. I ordered fresh tea and we sat and talked till it was dark. Little did I think that this meeting would turn my little world upside down. Things would never be the same again.

I could speak many languages, having been home-taught: French, English, Ceylonese. I said that perhaps this might help the war effort as I couldn't leave the farm so it was agreed that a wireless station should be set up. I was to become a spy for the British army, to relay reports of ships or aircraft and movements of troops as and when. This sounded fun, but how mistaken I was as all too soon I had been recruited into training my men in sabotage, to destroy the railway from Rangoon to Myithina, the last stop of the line to India.

The army supplied us with a rifle apiece and a hand gun, and boxes of dynamite and fuses, and a map, and said, *Take your men and go down and destroy this railway line, to stop the Jap troops reaching India.* I was not given a choice: it was an order, leaving me little time to arrange the care of my lovely tea plantation. Harvest picking had been done and sent off to the exporters. So, choosing the older of the experienced men to stay behind, I left them in charge, with instructions that if anything did happen to me, I could not see that far ahead, the farm would be theirs. I took the young men who wanted to go.

My farm was set high above the tree line with far-reaching views out to sea some hundred miles away. With only a map we moved down over rivers and through the dense jungle until we sat on a bank overlooking the rails. We discussed what we should do. Spark was with me, like a black shadow. We slid down to the line, hoping that we could set the dynamite before the train came. I lay down and put my ear to the line to see if I could feel the vibrations of a train: nothing yet. Good – we had time.

The men worked quickly and quietly. I was proud of my boys. We laid four lots along the track when suddenly Spark began to growl: he had heard something I had not. Fuses set and wired up to the plunger, I signalled them to climb the bank, taking the dog with them. I was left to press the plunger. With the sound of the train coming, I hid myself far enough away for safety, I thought, and waited for the train. I had to make sure that the train had passed the first lot so they could not retreat. I waited, holding my breath. The train was full of Japs, some riding on the footplate of the engine. This was the fourth time we had blown the trains up but they still seemed to come.

I pushed the plunger down and the explosion was so great the train was thrown up into the air. With the brakes screeching, shouts and screams of the men, the train rolled down the hillside into the river below. All in a flash, I lost my footing and fell backwards as the third explosion went off. They were set a few seconds apart. As I lay with my heavy bag on my back, the explosion burst my eardrums and blew me apart. As I was flying through the air in the last seconds of life, thoughts whizzed through my mind as a memory of life. How stupid of me to be blown to bits. I had trained the boys about this very same thing – what not to do.

This particular part was known as Hell Pass and this is where my life ended.

My name was Harry, named after my grandfather in England. I was short with a mass of thick, black hair and brown eyes. I was very much like my Ceylon side of the family. My skin was not white but neither of my parents had white skin. Father, although somewhere along the family line came from white British, his mother had also been Ceylonese.

I died on 19th July 1943, aged 39.

Harry

NB: Hell Fire Pass was between Burma and India. The Japs were building a rail road, using prisoners of war to do the work, which was destroyed by locals behind and down the line. This bloody war claimed hundreds of lives. Prisoners who were too weak to work were shot and others took their place. Little was known about people like Harry who gave up their farms and plantations to help the British fight the war against the Japanese invasion.

Received 7th March 2007.

Gurkha Soldier 1943

My name is Rani and I am a Gurkha serving with the Gurkha Rifles in the British Army in Burma. I am a corporal, of no high rank but I am a proud man. Part of my equipment is my kukri: it's more important than my rifle for my life's protection. I am small in size. We are all much shorter than the British soldiers. Although I am short, it does not make any difference to how I fight – the Gurkhas are known for their bravery and fierceness.

I don't speak your English language but Gurklie. My home is a small place outside Kathmandu. My uncle is a Buddhist monk but most of my family are dead. But Fate made me a soldier. I was called to fight at the age of 18. I cannot read or write but my knowledge of the world around me is good. I know every bird by its song, every flower and tree, and I love music.

As a child, I would climb the mountain and go to the monastery in Nepal where my uncle lived. The air was crisp and cold. The click-clack of the prayer flags would cut through my mind and quicken my heart beat: it was a thrill just to be there. I think uncle would have liked me to have followed him but my eyes were set on far horizons. Now I had the chance to open up my small world.

I was walking into dense, dark jungle. We had to be alert now, no time to let your mind wander with childhood dreams. We were told to search out the Jap hideouts: these were tunnels running criss-cross under foot, so well hidden you could walk within two strides of it and not even see it. Talking was not allowed. Most communication was done with hand signals. But, if I was a Jap, I would hear anyone coming as we hacked our way through the tangled undergrowth with our kukries. It must have sounded like a herd of stampeding elephants.

It was humid and sticky, with swarms of biting insects plaguing our skin. The British soldier felt it worse, having fair skin. They did not worry me that much.

I longed for the crisp mountain air as it was not possible to breath this foul-smelling air filled with rotting vegetation.

Before we noticed, we had tripped a snare to a tunnel and all hell broke out. As we hit the ground and tried to take cover, firing started and three of my mates were hit and killed before my eyes. This was the first actual action that I had ever seen: no time to raise my rifle to return fire. I was shot in the stomach. I heard no more. Our platoon had lost four soldiers in one minute.

As I lay in my own blood, I noticed a tall man standing beside me. He was all in white. I thought that he was a monk. Bending down, he took my hand and pulled me to my feet. He said little but I knew his thoughts. So strange that I felt no more pain, and as I rose, my mates followed.

Then we seemed to float above the ground. The stranger still held my hand. Far above the jungle we flew. I can't explain it any other way. Then I saw the mountains of Nepal below me. I was at the top, looking down. I could see the prayer flags in all their bright colours but I could not hear them. Monks were but little dots and I knew that uncle would never see me again, but I did not worry.

Life was not at an end, the stranger told me, not in words but in through thoughts. This was a start of a new life and adventures for me that would bring much happiness. No more death or sorrow but the meeting up with my family again.

I had a bit of a problem. I was told to contact you but if I spoke to you, you wouldn't understand me so I was given a soul who could translate my words so this is how I came to you.

Thank you for your thoughts and healing that you have given to me.

Rani

Received 23/01/2007

Remember Me
(The voice of the dead)

Remember me
Duty called and I went to war
Though I'd never fired a gun before
I paid the price for your new day
As all my dreams were blown away

Remember me
We all stood true as whistles blew
And faced the shell and stench of Hell
Now battle's done, there is no sound
Our bones decay beneath the ground
We cannot see, or smell, or hear
There is no death, or hope or fear

Remember me
Once we, like you, would laugh and talk
And run and walk and do the things that you all do
But now we lie in rows so neat
Beneath the soil, beneath your feet

Remember me
In mud and gore and the blood of war
We fought and fell and move no more
Remember me, I am not dead
I'm just a voice within your head

Harry Riley

Regrets

The thing I regret most of all as I lay dying of shrapnel wounds was that I would never hold my wife or child in my arms again. Derek was five years old when I left for war, in 1943, out to Tripoli on a troop ship. Hundreds of us went. Somewhere on the quayside stood my little family. I could not see them. I searched the crowds, panicking that we would sail before I could wave goodbye. When I did spot them, the boat was pulling away from the dock. I waved and blew kisses and they saw me. Tears blinded me: I was glad they did not see this. I knew, I just knew that I would not see them again, but all the same I called, *I'll be home, sweetheart!*

My name was Keith and I was 29. Before the war I was a reporter come newspaper typesetter and the paper had asked me to go as the news correspondent, reporter. I lived in Worcestershire.

I was needed to relay news from the front line the British Empire expects you to do your best. Reports were sent home whenever possible, usually by telegram. This way, I was permitted to enter a few cryptic words for my wife. Although I never heard from her, I knew I was in their prayers every night. Derek and I had been very close as a father and son were. He was good at kicking a ball and he had endless energy, more than I had. He often left me panting for breath.

My line of work gave me little exercise as I sat at a desk all day. This exercise would not help me on the long marching that lay ahead of me through the scorching sands of north Africa. I took a long time to die so had plenty of time to remember the little things that gave us joy: walking on the Clent Hills, the green fields and small country lanes round the small hamlet under the shadow of the Clent Hills.

I had just sent my report in when suddenly my world was turned upside down. A blinding flash and everything went black as a mortar exploded close to where I was sitting, and I was torn apart. I lay in my own blood as life seeped away. I felt a medic touch my neck, looking for a pulse. My strong heartbeat was now fluttering liked a trapped butterfly, and the words, the last I ever heard, *Leave him, he has gone.*

But I was still alive, on the edge of death, but the little spark of life was still there.

My soul was still inside me but now the light was so bright and I found myself floating above the ground. How could this be? A small hand slipped into mine, a child, about the same age as Derek, and I was whisked away. I was asked if there was anywhere I would like one more look at. I said, *Home, please,* and I was there, standing as a young boy again on the Clent Hills among the bracken and the yellow gorse alive with bees. Then I was gone again.

I passed to the bright world just a few days before my 30th birthday. It was the 15th September 1944.

Thank you for helping me forward.

Keith.

Received 7/5/2007

Ian Tick Fever

Hallo, I am Ian. I am 22 years old. My home is in Broadway in the Cotswolds. I am of medium build with carrot-red hair and green eyes and covered with freckles. My nickname at school was Carrots. I suppose anyone with my fair colouring would doubtless get teased.

I am in a POW camp near Tripoli in north Africa, caught and put here at the beginning of the war when the plane I flew was shot down, along with the rest of the crew that lived.

With my fair complexion and no shelter, I am terribly burned. Large, deep, festering burns cover my body, infested by flies. My mates try to wash the sores with salty water but with no real result. But worst of all are the fleas and ticks in the desert sands. Men are dying every day from tick fever.

Our German guards have no pity for us as we try to erect small areas of shade for the sickest men.

The sun is relentless. I am dreaming of the gentle spring rain and the days when endless rain stopped the cricket matches on the England's green and pleasant land. I made myself a promise never again to complain when it rained.

Days and nights drag on. Some men have gone blind. We are kept short of water to drink and can't wash to keep our sores clean. We are all under nourished and dirty while outside the barbed wire the Germans shower every day, taunting us by throwing away fresh water. No Red Cross parcels from home. I would do anything for the clean smell of soap.

Tick fever is taking men every day. I know that my time is running out, as even in the hottest part of the day I am shivering out of control. In the darkest hours of night, why is it that I am the only one to see flashes of bright colours? I am lying outside under the stars to keep cool. Living under canvas is unbearable: we can't breathe. I dream it's raining. I can smell new-cut grass. I am sitting in the meadow under the tree I loved to climb when I was 9 years old on the edge of the bluebell woods. I can hear the cuckoo calling and the sound of a cricket ball on willow. Memories are all I have left now. I can't remember why I am here let alone my rank and number. All reason for living anymore has been washed away in pain and suffering.

British planes fly over daily, and rumours say that the British front lines are gaining ground. Will they rescue us soon? Sorry – I seem to have rambled on. I long to be set free but I know that only death will set me free.

Ian died of tick fever on 20th August 1944.

Received 22nd August 2009

Hospital Ship

I never thought anyone would hear my thoughts. I have never for one moment forgotten my loved ones back home. I've been over here a long time with no one to console me or help me forget the horrors of war.

I am Mary, 26 years old, a nurse with the Queen Alexander's nurses. I trained at King's College Hospital in 1937. I joined the navy in peacetime to see the world but I did not get as far as I wanted to as war broke out in 1939, and I sailed for the far east. I loved my life before the war and rubbing shoulders with all the crew, the dances and the fun, and so many captured young men. Life was really good in the years before the war. Life would never be the same again, alas.

We sailed to Aden first and then onto Hong Kong where our troops were in combat against the Japs. Our ship became a floating hospital and carried a large Red Cross flag which was flying all the time. Also, the emblem was painted on the deck and funnels so there was no excuse for not recognising us under the Geneva Convention which proclaimed that any hospital ship should not be under fire from any side. But unfortunately, the Japs did not have any care about anyone flying the Red Cross flag. We were in British waters but it made no difference.

We had loaded up with the worst lot of injuries which needed more treatment than we could do. We had been at sea for two days when the watch crew spotted a swarm of black planes zooming down on us. Our guns were always primed ready but so far we had not employed them in war but now we were under attack. Bombing the ship, again and again, then torpedoes were dropped. We were hopelessly outnumbered and did not stand a chance.

Our sailors put up a brave fight with our anti-aircraft guns, hitting one or two, but not enough to save our ship. They were ruthless, firing at all on deck, even dive bombing us by flying into the ship in a suicide dive. We had never seen so much hatred in our lives. Later, they were known as Kamikaze pilots. All the time, a rush against how long the ship would stay afloat. We tried to rescue the worst injured into life boats.

It was useless as if anyone got off, they would be hopelessly unprotected against them. The ship's crew fought bravely but we were sinking fast.

I was below decks trying to reassure the wounded that we would be saved, knowing all the time it was not true. A torpedo hit below the waterline and the cabins were filling up with water. I was up to my neck now. Those on the bunks were under water, drowning or already dead. Equipment and boxes were floating round my face. I was struggling to keep my nose out of the water, fighting for my life, when suddenly something hit my head and I slipped under thewater. Then the ship went down.

I found myself dry and sitting on a bench, don't know where or how I got there. My thoughts turned to my family back at home. Before I left for sea in 1939, my little sister gave birth to a little girl. Her sister had been killed in France at the beginning of the war and she took it all so hard. I had promised that I would come home and look after her and my God child but I have failed her and I am so sorry. This is something I could never forgive myself for.

Until you heard me calling you, I now know that I had no choice of when I should live or die. I can now come to terms and stop being so angry. Being angry and bitter has stopped me from letting go of things that were out of my control and get on with my spirit life.

Thank you, a true friend you are to those in need.

Bless you.

Mary

Received 8/4/2008

74

They went with songs into the battle, they were young,
Straight of limb, true of eye, steady and aglow.
They were staunch to the end against odds uncounted,
They fell with their faces to the foe.

They shall not grow old, as we that are left grow old:
Age shall not weary them, nor the years condemn.
At the going down of the sun and in the morning
We will remember them.

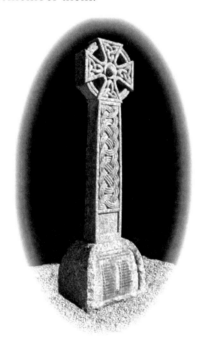

The Kohima Epitaph

**When you go home, tell them of us and say
For your tomorrow we gave our today.**